INTERMITTENT FASTING FOR WOMEN OVER 50

The Ultimate Guide to Improve Health and Longevity

Donna R. Williams

TABLE OF CONTENT

INTRODUCTION

Racheal had always been an active person, but as she reached her 50s, she started to feel her age more and more. She was overweight and had high blood pressure and cholesterol. She knew she needed to make a change to get healthier, but she wasn't sure where to begin.

One day she was watching a documentary about intermittent fasting and how it could help people lose weight and improve their overall health. She was intrigued, so she decided to give it a try.

At first, she was nervous about the idea of not eating for extended periods of time, but she soon found that it wasn't as hard as she thought it would be. She began to stick to a 16-hour fast with an 8-hour eating window. During her eating window, she focused on eating healthy and nutritious foods.

With time, Racheal started to see the results of her new lifestyle. She lost weight and her blood pressure and cholesterol levels returned to normal. She also felt more energized and had more clarity in her mind.

Racheal was so pleased with the results that she continued intermittent fasting even after she met her goals. She ended up feeling healthier than she had in decades and was able to maintain her weight and health even as she got older.

Racheal had finally found a way to live a healthy life after 50 and she was thrilled. She would recommend intermittent fasting to anyone looking to improve their health and wellbeing.

Intermittent fasting is an increasingly popular dieting strategy that has become a go-to for many individuals over the age of 50. It is a flexible approach to eating that allows individuals to eat within a specific window of time, with periods of fasting in between. This type of fasting has been around for centuries, but has recently become more popular due to its potential health benefits.

Intermittent fasting can be an especially beneficial dieting strategy for women over 50, as it can help promote weight loss, reduce inflammation, and improve overall health. It can also help to increase energy levels and reduce stress levels, making it a great option for those looking to improve their overall health and well-being.

In this book, we will examine the benefits of intermittent fasting for women over 50, as well as how to properly utilize this dieting strategy to achieve optimal health results. We will discuss the different types of intermittent fasting, how to customize the approach to fit individual needs, and the potential risks and side effects associated with this type of dieting. We will also provide some tips on how to make the most out of intermittent fasting and how to integrate it into a healthy lifestyle.

By the end of this book, readers will have a better understanding of the potential health benefits of intermittent fasting, as well as how to safely and effectively incorporate this dieting approach into their daily lives. The goal is to provide readers with the tools and information they need to make informed decisions about their health and to achieve their goals in a safe and sustainable fashion.

CHAPTER 1

What is Intermittent Fasting?

An eating habit known as intermittent fasting cycles between periods of eating and fasting. It does not specify which foods you should eat, but rather when you should eat them. It is a popular weight-loss method that has been gaining a lot of attention in recent years.

Intermittent fasting has a variety of health benefits, including improved mental clarity, increased energy levels, weight loss, and improved metabolic health. It is also thought to help regulate hormones, decrease inflammation, and reduce the risk of certain diseases.

Cycles of fasting and eating occur frequently during intermittent fasting. During the fasting period, you typically eat nothing or very few calories. During the eating period, you can eat whatever you want. This cycle can be done in many different ways, including daily, weekly, or monthly.

Intermittent fasting can be a great way to start a healthier lifestyle. It is important to remember, however, that it is not a miracle cure and should be done in combination with a healthy and balanced diet and an exercise regimen. As with any diet or lifestyle change, it is important to talk to your doctor before you start.

Intermittent fasting is a great way to jumpstart your health journey and take control of your life. With a combination of a healthy diet and exercise, intermittent fasting can help you reach your health and fitness goals

Intermittent fasting is a dietary pattern that cycles between periods of fasting and eating. It has become a popular weight-loss plan, and many studies have found that it can be beneficial for overall health. Women over 50 may be particularly interested in this plan, as a way to stay healthy, lose weight, and even slow down the aging process.

The most common type of intermittent fasting is called the 16/8 method, which involves fasting for 16 hours and eating within an 8-hour window. This can be done every day, or just a few days a week. For example, one could fast from 6 pm to 10 am each day, and then eat two meals within the 8-hour window. This is a good option for those who want to make fasting a part of their daily routine.

Women over 50 should understand that fasting may not be the best option for them. As we age, our bodies become more sensitive to fasting, and it can be more difficult to maintain the plan. Additionally, fasting can cause hormonal imbalances, which can be particularly problematic for women. If you are a woman over 50 and considering intermittent fasting, it is important to consult with a doctor before beginning the plan.

Women over 50 should also be aware of the potential risks of fasting. Fasting can cause dehydration, fatigue, and headaches. Additionally, fasting can lead to excessive weight loss, which can be dangerous for older women. It is important to monitor your weight and ensure that you are eating enough to meet your body's needs.

Intermittent fasting can be a great tool for weight loss and overall health, but it is important for women over 50 to understand the potential risks before beginning a plan. It is best to speak with a doctor before starting an intermittent fasting plan to make sure it is a safe option for you.

In conclusion, intermittent fasting can be a great option for weight loss and overall health for women over 50. However, it is important to understand the potential risks and to consult with a doctor before beginning a plan. With proper guidance, intermittent fasting can be a safe and effective way to stay healthy and lose weight.

CHAPTER 2

Benefits of Intermittent Fasting for Women Over 50

Intermittent fasting is a popular trend among dieters of all ages, but it may offer special benefits for women over 50. While intermittent fasting can help to reduce body weight and improve metabolic health, it also has unique benefits for women over 50. This chapter will explore the potential benefits of intermittent fasting for women over 50, including weight loss, improved metabolic health, increased energy levels, and improved cognitive function.

Weight Loss: Intermittent fasting can help women over 50 to achieve their weight loss goals. By reducing caloric intake, intermittent fasting can help to reduce body fat and body weight. This can be beneficial for women who have experienced difficulty losing weight in the past.

Improved Metabolic Health: Intermittent fasting can also improve metabolic health. By reducing caloric intake, intermittent fasting can help to lower blood glucose levels, reduce insulin resistance, and reduce cholesterol levels. This can be beneficial for women over 50 who are at risk for metabolic diseases such as type 2 diabetes and heart disease.

Increased Energy Levels: Intermittent fasting can also increase energy levels. By reducing caloric intake, intermittent fasting can reduce fatigue and help to improve overall energy levels. This can be beneficial for women over 50 who often experience fatigue and low energy levels.

Improved Cognitive Function: Intermittent fasting can also help to improve cognitive function. By reducing caloric intake, intermittent fasting can help to improve memory, focus, and concentration. This can be beneficial for women over 50 who may be experiencing age-related cognitive decline.

In conclusion, intermittent fasting can offer many potential benefits for women over 50. By reducing caloric intake, intermittent fasting can help to reduce body weight, improve metabolic health, increase energy levels, and improve cognitive function. For women over 50, intermittent fasting can be a safe and effective way to achieve their weight loss goals and improve their overall health.

CHAPTER 3

Potential Risks of Intermittent Fasting for Women Over 50

Intermittent fasting is an increasingly popular dietary trend that has been linked to a variety of health benefits, including weight loss and improved metabolic health. While intermittent fasting may provide some benefits for some people, it is important to be aware of the potential risks and side effects of this dietary approach, especially for women over 50. This chapter will discuss the potential risks and side effects of intermittent fasting for women over 50, and provide advice for minimizing these risks.

1. **Nutritional Deficiencies**: One of the most common risks associated with intermittent fasting is the potential to develop nutritional deficiencies. Women over 50 are particularly vulnerable to nutritional deficiencies due to their increased risk of osteoporosis, anemia, and other age-related conditions. Therefore, it is important for women over 50 to ensure that they are consuming adequate amounts of essential nutrients, such as calcium, iron, and B vitamins, when practicing intermittent fasting.

2. **Dehydration:** Dehydration is another potential risk associated with intermittent fasting. Due to the reduced intake of food, it is

important to ensure that adequate amounts of water are consumed throughout the day. Furthermore, it is important to note that caffeine has a diuretic effect and can increase the risk of dehydration. Therefore, women over 50 should limit their caffeine intake when intermittent fasting.

3. Muscle Loss: Intermittent fasting can also lead to muscle loss due to inadequate protein intake. Women over 50 are particularly vulnerable to muscle loss, as age-related muscle loss is more pronounced in older individuals. Therefore, it is important to ensure that adequate amounts of protein are consumed when intermittent fasting to minimize the risk of muscle loss.

4. Low Energy Levels: Lastly, intermittent fasting can lead to low energy levels due to the reduced food intake. This can make it more difficult for women over 50 to complete everyday activities and can lead to feelings of fatigue. To minimize this risk, it is important to ensure that adequate amounts of healthy carbohydrates are consumed throughout the day.

In conclusion, intermittent fasting can provide some benefits for some people, however, it is important to be aware of the potential risks and side effects of this dietary approach, especially for women over 50. By following the advice provided in this chapter, women over 50 can minimize the risks associated with intermittent fasting and maximize the potential benefits.

Implementing Intermittent Fasting

Intermittent fasting is a popular and growing lifestyle trend that is gaining traction among health-conscious individuals. It involves alternating between periods of eating and fasting, usually for 16-24 hours at a time. This can be done in a variety of ways, such as restricting yourself to one to two meals per day, fasting for 24 hours once or twice a week, or even fasting for multiple days at a time. It is important to note that intermittent fasting is not a diet, but rather a pattern of eating that has been found to have many health benefits.

We will discuss how to successfully implement intermittent fasting into your lifestyle. We will also discuss some potential benefits and risks associated with intermittent fasting. Finally, we will provide some tips and advice to get the most out of your intermittent fasting experience.

1. Choose the Right Protocol

There are several different intermittent fasting protocols that you can choose from. It is important to choose the right protocol for your lifestyle and goals. The most well-known protocols are the 16/8, 5:2, and alternate-day fasting regimens.

The 16/8 protocol involves fasting for 16 hours and eating during an 8-hour window. This is often done by skipping breakfast and eating all of your meals during the afternoon and evening.

The 5:2 protocol involves eating normally for 5 days of the week and then fasting for 2 days. During the fasting days, you can either fast completely or eat very little.

Alternate day fasting involves fasting for 24 hours and then eating normally for the next 24 hours.

2. Set Realistic Goals

Before you start implementing intermittent fasting, it is important to set realistic goals. You should also take into account any health conditions or medications you are taking. It is important to consult with your doctor before starting any new diet or lifestyle change.

Once you have set your goals and consulted with your doctor, you can start to plan out your meals and fasting periods.

3. Start Slowly

It is important to start slowly when implementing intermittent fasting. Start with shorter fasting windows, such as 14 or 16 hours, and gradually work your way up to longer ones. This will help your body adjust to the change and reduce the risk of experiencing any negative side effects.

You should also make sure to stay hydrated and get enough sleep during your fasting periods.

4. Eat Nutrient-Dense Foods

During your eating window, it is important to focus on eating nutrient-dense and unprocessed foods. Eating a variety of whole foods, such as fruits, vegetables, lean proteins, and healthy fats, will provide you with the essential nutrients your body needs.

It is also important to avoid processed and sugary foods, as these can lead to an increased risk of developing chronic diseases.

5. Monitor Your Progress

Finally, it is important to monitor your progress. This can be done by keeping track of your weight, energy levels, and overall health. If you experience any negative side effects, such as fatigue, headaches, or light headedness, then you may need to adjust your fasting protocol.

Intermittent fasting can be a useful tool for weight loss and overall health, but it is important to remember that it is not a miracle cure. When implemented properly and combined with a healthy diet and lifestyle, intermittent fasting can be a great way to improve your health and reach your goals.

We hope this chapter has provided you with useful information on how to successfully implement intermittent fasting into your lifestyle. Now that you have a better understanding of the basics, you can start to experiment and find out which methods work best for you.

CHAPTER 4

Strategies for Successful Intermittent Fasting

Intermittent fasting can be a powerful tool for achieving your health and wellness goals, but it is not a one-size-fits-all approach. Everyone's body is different and has different needs, so it's important to tailor your intermittent fasting strategy to work best for you. In this chapter, we'll explore some of the ways you can make intermittent fasting work for you.

First, it's important to choose an intermittent fasting schedule that fits your lifestyle. Some of the most popular intermittent fasting schedules are the 16/8 method, the 5:2 diet, and the alternate-day fasting. Each of these methods has its own unique benefits, so take some time to consider which one would be best for you.

Second, it's important to choose the right foods to eat during your fasting period. When it comes to intermittent fasting, it's important to focus on nutrient-dense, whole foods like fruits, vegetables, nuts, seeds, and lean proteins. Eating nutrient-dense foods will help ensure that your body is getting the nutrients it needs while you're fasting.

Third, it's important to stay hydrated. Staying hydrated is essential for good health and it's even more important when you're fasting. Make sure to drink plenty of water throughout your fasting period. Additionally, you can also drink calorie-free beverages like herbal teas and sugar-free drinks to help keep you hydrated and feeling satisfied.

Finally, it's important to keep track of your progress. Intermittent fasting can be a powerful tool for achieving your health and wellness goals, but it's important to track your progress to ensure that you're staying on track. Consider keeping a journal or using an app to help you monitor your progress.

Intermittent fasting can be a great way to achieve your health and wellness goals, but it's important to customize it to best suit your needs. By choosing the right intermittent fasting schedule, eating the right foods, staying hydrated, and tracking your progress, you can make intermittent fasting work for you.

Working Out While Fasting

A lot of people wonder about working out while fasting? Is it possible to exercise while fasting, and if so, what are the benefits? This chapter will explore the potential benefits and drawbacks of working out during intermittent fasting, as well as the ways in which it can be done safely and effectively.

The Benefits of Working Out During Intermittent Fasting

Many people report feeling more energized and alert when they work out during fasting periods. This is likely due to the fact that when fasting, your body is able to access stored energy more quickly, providing a surge of energy for your workout. Additionally, working out during a fast can help to support increased fat burning, as your body is more likely to use stored fat for energy rather than carbohydrates.

In addition to the fat-burning benefits, working out during intermittent fasting can also help to boost your mental clarity and focus. When your body is in a fasted state, it is better able to access and use stored energy, resulting in improved concentration and focus during your workout.

Finally, working out during intermittent fasting can help to increase the effectiveness of your workouts. When your body is in a fasted state, it is more sensitive to the effects of exercise, resulting in an increased response to the stimulus of the workout.

Drawbacks of Working Out During Intermittent Fasting

There are some drawbacks to working out during intermittent fasting as well. Since your body is not taking in food, it is more likely to become fatigued during the workout, resulting in a lower intensity workout. Additionally, since your body is not taking in any nutrients, it is more likely to experience muscle soreness and fatigue after the workout.

Finally, working out during intermittent fasting can increase the risk of dehydration, as your body is not taking in any fluids. This can be especially problematic if you are engaging in high-intensity exercise.

Tips for Working Out During Intermittent Fasting

If you decide to work out during a fast, there are several tips that can help you to do so safely and effectively. First, it is important to stay hydrated throughout your fast, as this can help to reduce the risk of dehydration and fatigue. Additionally, you should make sure to keep your workouts relatively low intensity, as your body is likely to become fatigued more quickly.

Finally, it is important to make sure that you break your fast with a meal that is high in protein and healthy fats. This will help to replenish your energy stores and support muscle growth and recovery.

Working out during intermittent fasting can have several potential benefits, including increased fat burning and improved mental clarity and focus. However, there are some drawbacks as well, including increased risk of dehydration and fatigue. If you decide to work out during a fast, make sure to stay hydrated and keep your workouts relatively low intensity. Additionally, make sure to break your fast with a meal that is high in protein and healthy fats. By following these tips, you can safely and effectively work out during intermittent fasting.

CHAPTER 5

What to Eat During Intermittent Fasting

Intermittent fasting is a popular lifestyle practice that can help you lose weight, improve your overall health, and more. However, choosing the right foods to eat during intermittent fasting is essential for achieving the best results.

This chapter will provide an overview of the different types of foods to eat during intermittent fasting. We'll also discuss a few tips to help you make the most of your fasting period.

Types of Foods to Eat During Intermittent Fasting

When it comes to intermittent fasting, you'll want to choose foods that are nutrient-dense and filling. This will help you feel satiated and energized during your fasting period. Here are some of the best types of foods to eat during intermittent fasting:

-High-fiber fruits and vegetables: Fruits and vegetables are full of vitamins, minerals, and fiber, making them a great choice for an intermittent fasting diet. Choose a variety of colorful, nutrient-dense produce to get the most out of your fasting period.

-Lean proteins: Lean proteins, such as chicken, fish, and eggs, are a great source of energy and can help you feel full for longer. Choose lean cuts of meat and trim off any visible fat before cooking.

-High-fiber grains: High-fiber grains, such as quinoa, oats, and barley, are a great source of complex carbohydrates and fiber. They can help keep you feeling full and energized during your fasting period.

-Healthy fats: Healthy fats, such as olive oil, avocados, and nuts, can provide you with an additional source of energy and help you feel full for longer. Choose unsaturated fats over saturated ones.

-Low-sugar beverages: Low-sugar beverages, such as green tea, can help keep you hydrated and energized during your fasting period. Choose unsweetened varieties to avoid added sugar.

Tips for Making the Most of Your Intermittent Fasting Period

Making the most of your intermittent fasting period is key to achieving the best results. Here are a few tips to help you get the most out of your fasting period:

-Eat nutrient-dense foods: Eating nutrient-dense foods, such as those listed above, can help keep you feeling full and energized during your fasting period.

-Remain hydrated: Your body needs water to function correctly, so make sure you're getting plenty of it.

-Focus on quality, not quantity: During your fasting period, focus on eating high-quality, nutrient-dense foods rather than overeating.

-Get plenty of sleep: Getting enough sleep is essential for maintaining good health and energy levels during your fasting period. Aim to get at least 7-8 hours of sleep each night.

-Listen to your body: When it comes to intermittent fasting, it's important to listen to your body. If you're feeling overly hungry or tired, it may be time to adjust your fasting schedule.

By following these tips, you can maximize the benefits of your intermittent fasting diet and achieve the best results.

Intermittent fasting is a popular lifestyle practice that can help you lose weight, improve your overall health, and more. However, choosing the right foods to eat during intermittent fasting is essential for achieving the best results. This chapter provided an overview of the different types of foods to eat during intermittent fasting, as well as some tips to help you make the most of your fasting period. With the right combination of nutrient-dense foods, hydration, and quality sleep, you can maximize the benefits of intermittent fasting and achieve the best results.

CHAPTER 6

Meal Planning Tips for Intermittent Fasting

If you're considering intermittent fasting, meal planning is key. It can help you stay on track and make sure you're getting the right nutrition you need. Here are some meal planning tips for intermittent fasting:

1. Choose Your Meal Plan Wisely

Before you start any kind of meal plan, it's important to do your research and decide which plan is best for you. Different types of intermittent fasting plans involve different amounts of fasting, so make sure you understand the differences and choose a plan that works for you.

2. Create a Meal Schedule

Having a set meal schedule can help keep you on track and make sure you're getting all the nutrients you need. Don't forget to include snacks and drinks in your meal plan.

3. Prep Your Meals

Whether you're prepping meals for the week or just prepping them in advance, it can be a huge time saver. Try to plan out meals that are easy to make and require minimal effort.

4. Consume wholesome proteins and fats.

Healthy fats and proteins are important for maintaining your energy levels during intermittent fasting. Make sure you're getting enough of these nutrients by adding healthy fats and proteins to your meals.

5. Hydrate

Drinking plenty of water and other fluids throughout the day is essential for your health. Make sure you're drinking enough water and other fluids to stay hydrated and energized.

6. Eat Nutrient-Dense Foods

Intermittent fasting can be stressful on your body, so make sure you're getting enough nutrients by eating nutrient-dense foods. Try to include a variety of fruits, vegetables, and whole grains in your meals to make sure you're getting all the nutrients you need.

7. Track Your Progress

Tracking your progress can help you stay motivated and on track with your intermittent fasting plan. Keep track of what you're eating, how you're feeling, and any changes in your weight or energy levels.

Following these meal planning tips for intermittent fasting can help you stay on track and get the most out of your fasting plan. Remember to always consult with your doctor before starting any type of diet or exercise program.

Chapter 7

Managing Cravings While Fasting

While intermittent fasting can have many benefits, it can also be a challenge to manage cravings. This chapter will discuss strategies for managing cravings during intermittent fasting.

First, it is important to understand the physiological basis of hunger and cravings. Hunger is a normal physiological response to a lack of food, and cravings are a psychological response triggered by certain food cues or memories. The hormone ghrelin is released in response to hunger, and this hormone stimulates the appetite. Leptin is a hormone that is released in response to fullness, and this hormone signals to the brain that enough food has been eaten.

Intermittent fasting is a dieting approach in which periods of eating are alternated with periods of fasting. During the fasting period, hunger and cravings can be particularly strong. To manage these cravings, it is important to understand what types of foods and situations may trigger cravings. Common triggers for cravings include certain types of food, such as sweets or salty snacks, and certain situations, such as being around other people who are eating.

To manage cravings, it is important to have a plan in place to combat them. One strategy is to plan meals and snacks ahead of time so that hunger does not become overwhelming. It is also important to focus on eating nutrient-dense foods that will provide lasting energy and satisfaction. Additionally, engaging in activities that distract from cravings can be helpful. Examples of these activities include going for a walk, practicing mindfulness, or engaging in a hobby.

Another strategy to manage cravings is to understand the emotional triggers associated with them. Emotional eating can trigger cravings, so it is important to identify any patterns or triggers that may be associated with emotional eating. Once these triggers are identified, it can be helpful to use distraction techniques or to practice mindful eating to avoid overeating.

Finally, it is important to be aware of the potential risks of intermittent fasting, such as dehydration and nutrient deficiencies. If cravings become difficult to manage, it is important to consult a healthcare professional who can provide guidance and advice on how to best manage them.

In conclusion, managing cravings during intermittent fasting can be challenging, but it is possible with the right strategies. By planning meals and snacks ahead of time, focusing on nutrient-dense foods, engaging in activities that distract from cravings, understanding emotional triggers, and consulting a healthcare professional, it is possible to successfully manage cravings during intermittent fasting.

Staying Motivated

Intermittent fasting is a great tool to help you reach your health and fitness goals. However, it can be difficult to stay motivated during the process. This chapter will discuss some tips and strategies to help you stay motivated during intermittent fasting.

First, it is important to be realistic in your goals. Have a clear understanding of what your goals are and the timeline in which you want to achieve them. Set manageable goals that are achievable. This will help keep you motivated and on track.

Second, create a support system. Having a good support system can be incredibly helpful in staying motivated. Whether it is a friend, family member, or a group of like-minded individuals, having someone to talk to and encourage you along the way can be invaluable.

Third, take a break when needed. Intermittent fasting can be difficult and challenging. Taking a break from it once in a while can help refresh your motivation. This could be a day, a week, or even just a meal. Whatever it is, it can help keep you motivated.

Fourth, reward yourself. Celebrate your successes and milestones. This could be a special treat or a reward. Having something to look forward to can help keep you motivated in the long run.

Finally, remember why you are doing it. Reflect on your goals and why you decided to take on this challenge in the first place. It can help you stay motivated and focused.

These are just a few tips to help you stay motivated during intermittent fasting. With a clear goal in mind and a support system to help you, you can stay motivated and reach your goals.

Chapter 8

Overcoming Mental Barriers to Intermittent Fasting

When it comes to health and nutrition, the idea of intermittent fasting can be intimidating. After all, going without food for hours on end isn't exactly a pleasant prospect. But despite the initial discomfort, intermittent fasting has been shown to have numerous health benefits, both physical and mental. So why is it that so many people struggle to make the switch?

The answer lies in the mental barriers that prevent us from taking the plunge. These barriers can range from fear of hunger to feelings of guilt and shame associated with fasting. Understanding the various mental barriers and how to overcome them is essential if you want to successfully incorporate intermittent fasting into your lifestyle.

The first barrier to overcome is fear of hunger. Many people worry that going without food for extended periods of time will leave them feeling weak and lethargic.

Fortunately, this isn't the case. In fact, research has found that hunger is not a problem during intermittent fasting. People tend to adjust to the fasting schedule after a few days, and may even find that they have more energy throughout the day.

The second barrier is guilt and shame. There is a cultural stigma attached to fasting, with some people believing that it is a form of self-deprivation. This is not the case, however.

Intermittent fasting is actually a form of self-care. It can help to boost your metabolic rate, regulate your hormones, and improve your overall health.

The third barrier is the fear of success. Some people worry that if they are successful in incorporating intermittent fasting into their lifestyle, they won't be able to stick with it.

This is a common fear, but it is also unfounded. Intermittent fasting is a habit that can be adopted for life. With the right support and motivation, you can stick with it and reap the benefits for many years to come.

Finally, there is the fear of social judgement. Many people worry that if they start intermittent fasting, their friends and family will think they are crazy or unhealthy.

This is an understandable concern, but it is important to remember that the decision to embark on intermittent fasting is a personal one. People will ultimately respect your decision, and may even be inspired to follow suit.

By understanding the various mental barriers associated with intermittent fasting, you can take the necessary steps to overcome them. With the right mindset and support, you can successfully incorporate this lifestyle change into your everyday routine. This will enable you to reap the numerous health benefits associated with intermittent fasting and live a healthier, happier life.

Chapter 9

Building a Support Network

When it comes to intermittent fasting, having a strong support network is crucial for keeping yourself motivated and on track. It can be hard to go through the process on your own, so having a few people you can rely on to provide guidance and support can make a huge difference in your success.

In this chapter, we'll discuss how to reach out to others for support, including how to identify potential support networks and how to cultivate those relationships.

Identifying Potential Support Networks

The first step to building a support network during intermittent fasting is to identify potential support networks. Who are the people in your life who are likely to be understanding and supportive of your journey?

Think about family members, friends, colleagues, and even online communities. Are there any people in your life who have successfully completed an intermittent fasting program? If so, they may be a great resource for advice and encouragement.

Alternatively, you may want to join an online forum or Facebook group dedicated to intermittent fasting. Here, you can connect with others who are also following the same program as you, and you can share stories and tips.

Cultivating Relationships

Once you've identified potential support networks, the next step is to start cultivating relationships with those people. If you're reaching out to family and friends, let them know what you're doing and why you're doing it. Explain the benefits of intermittent fasting and how it can help you reach your health and fitness goals.

If you're joining an online forum or Facebook group, start participating in the conversations. Ask questions, share your experiences, and offer advice to others when you can. This will help you build relationships with the other members and gain their trust.

It's also important to be realistic about your expectations. Remember that you're asking these people for their support, not their approval. They may not understand why you're doing this, and that's okay. Just be patient and understanding and explain your reasons as best you can.

Finally, don't be afraid to reach out if you're feeling overwhelmed or discouraged. It's important to have someone you can turn to when things get tough. Just knowing that you have someone to talk to can make a huge difference in your motivation and determination to keep going.

Building a strong support network during intermittent fasting can be a major factor in your success. Identifying potential support networks and cultivating relationships with those people can help keep you motivated and on track. Remember to be patient, understanding, and realistic with your expectations, and don't be afraid to reach out if you need help. With the right support system in place, you'll be well on your way to achieving your health and fitness goals.

Chapter 10

Intermittent meal plan

Day 1:

Breakfast: Overnight oats with fresh berries and nuts

Ingredients:

-1/2 cup oats, old-fashioned

-half a cup almond milk (or any other type of milk)

a quarter cup plain Greek yogurt

1 tablespoon maple syrup or honey

a quarter cup fresh berries (any type you like)

-1 tbsp. chopped nuts (almonds, walnuts, or pecans)

Instructions:

1. Combine the oats, almond milk, yogurt, and honey or maple syrup in a small mixing bowl.

2. Wrap the bowl in plastic wrap and place it in the refrigerator overnight.

3. Remove the bowl from the refrigerator in the morning and toss in the fresh berries and chopped nuts.

4. Serve the oats cold or warm if desired in the microwave. Enjoy!

Lunch: Greek salad with grilled chicken and feta cheese

Ingredients

• 2 chicken breasts

• 2 cups romaine lettuce, chopped

• 1/4 cup red onion, thinly sliced

• 1/4 cup cucumber, diced

• 1/4 cup kalamata olives, pitted and sliced

• 1/4 cup feta cheese, crumbled

• 1/4 cup cherry tomatoes, halved

• 2 tablespoons olive oil

• 1 teaspoon garlic powder

• 1 teaspoon dried oregano

• 1/2 teaspoon black pepper

• 1/4 cup red wine vinegar

• 2 tablespoons lemon juice

Instructions

1. Preheat a grill to medium-high heat.

2. Season chicken breasts with garlic powder, oregano, black pepper, and 1 tablespoon of the olive oil.

3. Grill chicken breasts for 5-7 minutes per side, or until cooked through.

4. Remove from grill and let cool slightly before cutting into cubes.

5. In a large bowl, combine romaine lettuce, red onion, cucumber, kalamata olives, feta cheese, and cherry tomatoes.

6. In a small bowl, whisk together remaining olive oil, red wine vinegar, and lemon juice.

7. Pour dressing over salad and toss to combine.

8. Add grilled chicken cubes and toss once more.

9. Serve and enjoy!

Dinner: Baked salmon with roasted vegetables

Ingredients:

-4 (4-ounce) salmon fillets

-1/2 teaspoon olive oil

-1/2 teaspoon salt

-1/4 teaspoon ground black pepper

-1/4 teaspoon garlic powder

-1/4 teaspoon dried oregano

-1/4 teaspoon dried thyme

-1/4 teaspoon paprika

-1/4 teaspoon onion powder

-2 cups diced potatoes

-1 cup diced carrots

-1 cup diced zucchini

-2 tablespoons olive oil

-1/2 teaspoon salt

-1/4 teaspoon ground black pepper

-1/4 teaspoon garlic powder

Instructions:

1. Preheat oven to 400°F.

2. In a baking dish, place the salmon fillets. Brush each fillet with the olive oil, then season with the salt, pepper, garlic powder, oregano, thyme, paprika, and onion powder.

3. In a separate bowl, combine the potatoes, carrots, zucchini, olive oil, salt, pepper, and garlic powder. Toss until evenly coated.

4. Spread the vegetables around the salmon in the baking dish.

5. Bake for 20 minutes, or until the vegetables are tender and the salmon is cooked through.

6. Serve and enjoy.

Snack: Protein smoothie with banana and almond butter

Ingredients:

-1 banana

-1 scoop of whey protein powder

-1 tablespoon of almond butter

-1/2 cup of ice

-1/2 cup of almond milk

Instructions:

1. Peel and slice the banana.

2. Place the banana slices, protein powder, almond butter and almond milk in a blender.

3. Blend until smooth.

4. Add the ice and blend for a few seconds.

5. Pour the smoothie into a glass and enjoy!

Day 2:

Breakfast: Avocado toast with egg

Ingredients:

- 2 slices of toast (preferably whole grain)

- 1/2 of a ripe avocado

- 1 egg

- Salt and pepper to taste

- Optional: red pepper flakes

Instructions:

1. Preheat the oven to 400°F.

2. Toast the two slices of bread until they are faintly golden.

3. Peel and pit the avocado, then mash it in a bowl.

4. Spread the mashed avocado onto the two slices of toast.

5. Crack the egg into a small bowl and carefully slide it onto one of the slices of toast.

6. Place the two slices of toast on a baking sheet and bake in the oven for 10-12 minutes until the egg is cooked.

7. Remove from oven and season with salt, pepper, and optional red pepper flakes.

8. Serve and enjoy!

Lunch: Veggie wrap with hummus and tahini

Ingredients:

2 whole wheat tortillas

1/4 cup hummus

1/4 cup tahini

1/4 cup cooked quinoa

1/4 cup cooked black beans

1/2 cup diced tomatoes

1/4 cup diced red onion

1/4 cup crumbled feta cheese

1/4 cup chopped cucumber

1/4 cup chopped parsley

Instructions:

1. Preheat a large skillet over medium heat.

2. Spread each tortilla with a thin layer of hummus, followed by tahini.

3. Top each tortilla with quinoa, black beans, tomatoes, red onion, feta cheese, cucumber and parsley.

4. Carefully fold each tortilla in half, and place in the preheated skillet.

5. Cook for 3-4 minutes per side, or until golden brown and crispy.

6. Slice each wrap in half and serve. Enjoy!

Dinner: Zucchini noodles with pesto and grilled shrimp

Ingredients:

- 4 large zucchini

- 2 tablespoons olive oil

- 2 cloves garlic, minced

- Salt and pepper, to taste

- 1/2 cup pesto sauce

- 1 pound grilled shrimp, cooked and peeled

Preparation Time: 20 minutes

Instructions:

1. Using a spiralizer, spiralize the zucchini into noodles.

2. In a large skillet over medium-high heat, heat the olive oil. Add the zucchini noodles and garlic, season with salt and pepper. Cook, stirring occasionally, for 5-7 minutes until the noodles are tender.

3. Add the pesto sauce and stir to combine. Cook for another minute.

4. Cook for another 2-3 minutes, or until the grilled shrimp is heated through.

5. Serve the zucchini noodles with the grilled shrimp and pesto sauce. Enjoy!

Snack: Apple slices with peanut butter

Ingredients:

- 2 Apples

- 2 tablespoons of Peanut Butter

Instructions:

1. Wash the apples thoroughly and then slice them into small pieces.

2. Spread the peanut butter on top of the apple slices.

Day 3:

Breakfast: Chia seed pudding with fresh fruit

Ingredients:

- 3 tablespoons chia seeds

- 1 cup almond milk

- 1 teaspoon honey

- 1/4 teaspoon vanilla

- 1/4 cup fresh fruit (e.g. strawberries, blueberries, raspberries, etc.)

Instructions:

1. In a medium mixing bowl, combine the chia seeds, almond milk, honey, and vanilla extract.

2. Cover the bowl and place it in the fridge for at least two hours, or until the chia seeds have expanded and the mixture has thickened.

3. Once the chia seed pudding is ready, top it with the fresh fruit of your choice.

4. Serve chilled and enjoy!

Lunch: Quinoa bowl with roasted vegetables and grilled chicken

Ingredients:

1 cup quinoa

1 cup vegetable broth

1 bell pepper, sliced

1 onion, sliced

1 zucchini, cut into cubes

1/2 cup mushrooms, sliced

1/2 teaspoon garlic powder

1/2 teaspoon chili powder

1/4 teaspoon paprika

1/4 teaspoon dried oregano

1/4 teaspoon salt

1/4 teaspoon black pepper

2 tablespoons olive oil

1 chicken breast, grilled

Instructions:

1. Preheat oven to 425°F.

2. In a medium saucepan, bring the vegetable broth to a boil. Reduce the heat to low and add the quinoa. Cover and cook for 15 minutes.

3. Meanwhile, in a large bowl, combine the bell pepper, onion, zucchini, mushrooms, garlic powder, chili powder, paprika, oregano, salt, pepper, and olive oil. Toss to combine.

4. Spread the vegetables on a baking sheet. Bake for 20 minutes, stirring once halfway through.

5. Grill the chicken breast until cooked through.

6. To assemble the quinoa bowls, divide the quinoa among four bowls. Top with the roasted vegetables and grilled chicken. Enjoy!

Dinner: Roasted cauliflower and chickpea curry

Ingredients:

-1 head of cauliflower, chopped into florets

-1 can chickpeas, drained and rinsed

-1 tablespoon olive oil

-1 onion, diced

-3 cloves garlic, minced

-1 teaspoon ground coriander

-1 teaspoon ground cumin

-1 teaspoon ground ginger

-1 teaspoon turmeric

-1 teaspoon garam masala

-1 can (14 ounces) diced tomatoes

-1/2 cup coconut milk

-1/4 cup fresh cilantro chopped

-Salt and freshly ground black pepper, to taste

Instructions:

1. Preheat the oven to 400 degrees Fahrenheit. On a baking sheet, arrange cauliflower florets. Season with salt and pepper after drizzling with olive oil. 20–25 minutes, or until golden brown and soft.

2. Meanwhile, heat a large skillet over medium heat. Add onion and cook until softened, about 5 minutes. Add garlic, coriander, cumin, ginger, turmeric, and garam masala. Cook for 1 minute, stirring constantly.

3. Stir in chickpeas, tomatoes, and coconut milk. Bring to a simmer and cook for 5 minutes.

4. Add roasted cauliflower and cook for an additional 5 minutes.

5. Taste and adjust seasoning with salt and pepper, if needed.

6. Serve over cooked basmati rice, topped with fresh cilantro. Enjoy!

Snack: Greek yogurt with berries and chia seeds

Ingredients:

-1 cup Greek yogurt

-1/2 cup mixed berries (raspberries, blueberries, blackberries, etc.)

-2 tablespoons chia seeds

Instructions:

1. In a bowl, combine the Greek yogurt and mixed berries.

2. Stir the chia seeds into the yogurt and berry mixture.

3. Refrigerate the mixture for 30 minutes to allow the chia seeds to hydrate and thicken.

4. Serve the yogurt mixture chilled, garnished with extra berries, if desired. Enjoy!

Day 4:

Breakfast: Smoothie bowl with banana and almond milk

Ingredients:

-2 ripe bananas, peeled and frozen

-1 cup almond milk

-1 tablespoon honey

-1/2 teaspoon ground cinnamon

-1/4 teaspoon ground nutmeg

-1/4 teaspoon vanilla extract

-1/4 cup granola

-1/4 cup sliced almonds

-1/4 cup fresh or frozen berries

Instructions:

1. In a blender, combine the frozen bananas, almond milk, honey, cinnamon, nutmeg, and vanilla extract. Blend until smooth.

2. Pour the smoothie into a bowl.

3. Top with granola, sliced almonds, and berries.

4. Serve and enjoy!

Lunch: Lentil soup with grilled cheese sandwich

Ingredients

For the Soup:

- 1 cup of dried lentils

- 1 large onion, diced

- 2 cloves garlic, minced

- 2 carrots, diced

- 2 stalks celery, diced

- 2 tablespoons olive oil

- 1 teaspoon dried oregano

- 1 teaspoon ground cumin

- 4 cups vegetable broth

- Salt and pepper, to taste

For the Grilled Cheese Sandwich:

- 4 slices of your favorite bread

- 4 slices of cheese (cheddar, Swiss, etc.)

- 2 tablespoons butter, melted

Instructions

1. Heat the olive oil in a large soup pot over medium heat. Combine the onion, garlic, carrots, and celery in a mixing bowl. Cook for 5 minutes, or until the vegetables are softened.

2. Add the lentils, oregano, cumin and broth. Bring to a boil, then reduce the heat and simmer for 20 minutes, or until the lentils are tender.

3. Meanwhile, make the grilled cheese sandwiches. Heat a large skillet over medium heat and add the butter. Place two slices of

bread in the skillet and top each with one slice of cheese. Place the other two slices of bread on top and cook until golden brown, about 2 minutes per side.

4. When the lentils are done, season the soup with salt and pepper, to taste.

5. Serve the soup with the grilled cheese sandwiches. Enjoy!

Dinner: Veggie stir-fry with brown rice

Ingredients:

-1 cup of brown rice

-2 tablespoons extra-virgin olive oil

-1 onion, chopped

-1 red bell pepper, chopped

-1 yellow bell pepper, chopped

-2 carrots, chopped

-1 cup mushrooms, sliced

-2 cloves garlic, minced

-1 teaspoon fresh ginger, minced

-3 tablespoons low-sodium soy sauce

-1 teaspoon sesame oil

-1/2 cup frozen peas

-1/2 cup broccoli florets

Instructions:

1. Cook the brown rice according to package instructions.

2. Heat the olive oil in a large skillet over medium-high heat. Add the onion, bell peppers, carrots, and mushrooms, and sauté for 5 minutes.

3. Add the garlic and ginger, and sauté for 1 minute.

4. Add the soy sauce and sesame oil, and stir to combine.

5. Add the frozen peas and broccoli, and cook for 2-3 minutes until the vegetables are tender.

6. Serve the stir-fry over the cooked brown rice. Enjoy!

Snack: Handful of nuts and dried fruit

Ingredients:

-Handful of Mixed Nuts (e.g. almonds, walnuts, hazelnuts, etc.)

-Handful of Dried Fruit (e.g. raisins, cranberries, goji berries, etc.)

Preparation Time: 5 minutes

Instructions:

1. Place the nuts and dried fruit in a bowl.

2. Mix them together until they are evenly distributed.

3. Enjoy!

Day 5:

Breakfast: Avocado and egg scramble

Ingredients:

- 2 eggs

- 1/4 cup chopped onion

- 2 tablespoons butter

- 1/2 avocado, diced

- Salt and pepper, to taste

Instructions:

1. Heat a medium skillet over medium heat.

2. Add butter and chopped onion to the skillet and cook until onion is softened and lightly browned (about 3 to 4 minutes).

3. Crack eggs into a bowl and whisk until combined.

4. Pour eggs into the skillet and stir to combine with the butter and onion.

5. Add diced avocado to the skillet and stir to combine.

6. Cook, stirring occasionally, until eggs are cooked through (about 5 minutes).

7. Season with salt and pepper to taste.

8. Serve hot. Enjoy!

Lunch: Grilled turkey and vegetable wrap

Ingredients:

-1 lb ground turkey

-1 onion, diced

-1 bell pepper, diced

-1 zucchini, diced

-1 teaspoon garlic powder

-1 teaspoon oregano

-1 teaspoon paprika

-1/2 teaspoon ground cumin

-1/2 teaspoon chili powder

-salt and pepper, to taste

-2 tablespoons olive oil

-4-8 large tortillas

-1/2 cup shredded cheese

-salsa, guacamole, lettuce or other toppings (optional)

Instructions:

1. In a large bowl, mix together the ground turkey, diced onion, bell pepper, zucchini, garlic powder, oregano, paprika, cumin, chili powder, salt, and pepper.

2. Heat the olive oil in a large skillet over medium-high heat. Add the turkey mixture and cook, stirring occasionally, until the turkey is cooked through and the vegetables are tender, about 10 minutes.

3. Assemble the wraps: lay out a tortilla, top with a scoop of the turkey and vegetable mixture, shredded cheese, and any other desired toppings. Roll up the wraps and place them on the grill.

4. Grill the wraps for 4-5 minutes, flipping halfway through, until the tortillas are lightly browned and the cheese is melted.

5. Serve the grilled turkey and vegetable wraps warm with salsa, guacamole, lettuce, or other desired toppings. Enjoy!

Dinner: Baked salmon with roasted sweet potatoes

Ingredients

- 2 large sweet potatoes, peeled and cut into cubes

- 2 tablespoons olive oil

- 2 cloves garlic, minced

- 2 tablespoons fresh rosemary, chopped

- 2 tablespoons fresh thyme, chopped

- 4 (6-8 ounce) salmon fillets

- Salt and pepper to taste

Instructions

1. Preheat oven to 400°F.

2. Spread the sweet potatoes out on a baking pan. Drizzle with olive oil and season with garlic, rosemary, thyme, salt, and pepper. Toss to coat.

3. Roast in preheated oven for 20 minutes.

4. Place salmon fillets on top of sweet potatoes. Drizzle with remaining olive oil and season with salt and pepper.

5. Bake for another 15-20 minutes, or until the salmon is cooked through and flakes easily with a fork.

6. Serve warm. Enjoy!

Snack: Protein shake with banana and almond butter

Ingredients:

-1 banana

-1 scoop of your favorite vanilla protein powder

-1 tablespoon of almond butter

-1/2 cup of almond milk

-1/4 cup of plain Greek yogurt

-1 teaspoon of honey

-1/4 teaspoon of ground cinnamon

-1/4 teaspoon of ground nutmeg

Instructions:

1. Combine the banana, protein powder, almond butter, almond milk, Greek yogurt, honey, cinnamon, and nutmeg in a blender.

2. Blend until the mixture is smooth and creamy.

3. Pour the protein shake into a glass and enjoy!

Day 6:

Breakfast: Oatmeal with fresh berries and nuts

Ingredients:

- 1 cup of oatmeal

- 2 cups of water

- 1/2 cup of fresh berries (blueberries, strawberries, or raspberries)

- 1/4 cup of chopped nuts (almonds, walnuts, or pecans)

- 2 tablespoons of honey or maple syrup (optional)

Instructions:

1. Bring water to a boil in a medium saucepan.

2. Add in the oatmeal and reduce heat to low. Cook for about 5 minutes, stirring occasionally.

3. Add in the berries and nuts, stirring to combine.

4. Cook for an additional 3-4 minutes, or until the oatmeal is cooked through and the berries and nuts are heated through.

5. Serve the oatmeal in individual bowls and add honey or maple syrup, if desired. Enjoy!

Lunch: Caesar salad with grilled chicken

Ingredients:

-2 boneless, skinless chicken breasts

-2 cloves of garlic, minced

-1 teaspoon of Italian seasoning

-1/4 cup of olive oil

-1/4 cup of freshly squeezed lemon juice

-2 heads of romaine lettuce, chopped

-1/2 cup of grated Parmesan cheese

-1/2 cup of croutons

-1/4 cup of Caesar salad dressing

Instructions:

1. Preheat the grill to medium-high heat.

2. Place the chicken breasts in a shallow dish and season with garlic, Italian seasoning, and a pinch of salt and pepper. Rub the seasoning into the chicken and let it sit for 10 minutes.

3. In a separate bowl, whisk together the olive oil and lemon juice. Brush the marinade over the chicken and let it sit for 10 minutes.

4. Place the chicken on the preheated grill and cook for 8-10 minutes, flipping halfway through, until the chicken is cooked through and the internal temperature has reached 165 degrees F.

5. Remove the chicken from the grill and let it rest for 5 minutes before slicing.

6. In a large bowl, combine the lettuce, Parmesan cheese, croutons, and Caesar dressing.

7. Slice the chicken and add to the salad. Toss to combine.

8. Serve the Caesar salad with grilled chicken immediately. Enjoy!

Dinner: Vegetarian quesadillas with black beans and corn

Ingredients:

- 4 Flour Tortillas

- 1 Can of Black Beans

- 1 Cup of Frozen Corn

- 1/2 Cup of Shredded Cheese

- 1/2 Cup of Chopped Onion

- 1/2 Cup of Chopped Bell Pepper

- 1/4 Cup of Sliced Olives

- 2 Tablespoons of Vegetable Oil

- 1/4 Teaspoon of Salt

- 1/4 Teaspoon of Ground Black Pepper

Instructions:

1. Heat the vegetable oil in a large skillet over medium heat.

2. Add the onions, bell peppers, and olives and cook for 5 minutes, stirring occasionally.

3. Add the corn and black beans and cook for an additional 5 minutes, stirring occasionally.

4. Remove the skillet from the heat and season with salt and pepper.

5. Place a tortilla in the skillet and sprinkle with one-fourth of the cheese and one-fourth of the bean-and-vegetable mixture.

6. Place a second tortilla on top and press down lightly.

7. Cook for 2 minutes, or until the bottom tortilla is lightly golden brown.

8. Flip the quesadilla and cook the other side for 2 minutes, or until lightly golden brown.

9. Remove the quesadilla from the skillet and place it onto a plate.

10. Repeat steps 5-9 with the remaining ingredients to make 3 more quesadillas.

11. Cut each quesadilla into 4 wedges and serve. Enjoy!

Snack: Kale chips

Ingredients:

-1 bunch of kale

-1 tablespoon olive oil

-Sea salt, to taste

Instructions:

1. Preheat oven to 350 degrees F.

2. Wash and dry the kale leaves, and then tear them into chip-sized pieces.

3. Place the kale in a large bowl and drizzle with olive oil.

4. Toss the kale to coat evenly.

5. Spread the kale onto a baking sheet in a single layer.

6. Sprinkle with sea salt.

7. Bake for 15 minutes, or until the kale is crisp and lightly browned.

8. Serve and enjoy!

Day 7:

Breakfast: Smoothie with banana, almond milk and spinach

Ingredients:

- 1 banana

- 1 cup almond milk

- 1 cup baby spinach

- 1 tablespoon honey (optional)

Instructions:

1. Peel and slice the banana.

2. Place the banana slices in a blender.

3. Add almond milk and baby spinach.

4. Blend until the mixture is smooth.

5. If desired, add honey to sweeten the smoothie.

6. Pour into a glass and enjoy!

Lunch: Lentil soup with grilled cheese sandwich

Ingredients

- 1 tablespoon olive oil

- 1 cup chopped onion

- 1 cup celery, diced

- 2 cloves garlic, minced

- 1 cup carrots, diced

- 2 cups lentils

- 6 cups vegetable broth

- 1 teaspoon dried thyme

- 1 bay leaf

- Salt and pepper, to taste

Grilled Cheese Sandwich:

- 4 slices bread

- 4 slices cheese

- 2 tablespoons butter

Instructions

1. Heat the olive oil in a large pot over medium heat. Add the onion, celery, garlic, and carrots and cook for about 5 minutes, stirring occasionally, until the vegetables are softened.

2. Add the lentils and vegetable broth to the pot. Stir in the thyme and bay leaf. Bring to a boil, then reduce the heat to low and simmer for about 25 minutes, until the lentils are tender.

3. Remove from heat and discard the bay leaf. Season with salt and pepper, to taste.

4. For the grilled cheese sandwich, butter one side of each slice of bread. Place two slices of bread, buttered-side-down, in a skillet over medium heat. Top each slice of bread with a slice of cheese, then top with the other two slices of bread, buttered-side-up.

5. Cook for about 3 minutes, until the bread is toasted and golden and the cheese is melted. Flip the sandwiches and cook for an additional 3 minutes, until the other side is toasted and golden.

6. Serve the lentil soup with the grilled cheese sandwiches. Enjoy!

Dinner: Grilled chicken with roasted vegetables

Ingredients:

-4 boneless, skinless chicken breasts

-1 teaspoon garlic powder

-1 teaspoon onion powder

-1 teaspoon paprika

-1 teaspoon dried oregano

-1 teaspoon dried thyme

-Salt and pepper, to taste

-2 tablespoons olive oil

-2 bell peppers, sliced

-1 red onion, sliced

-1 zucchini, sliced

-2 cloves garlic, minced

-2 tablespoons balsamic vinegar

Instructions:

1. Heat the grill on medium-high.

2. In a small bowl, mix together the garlic powder, onion powder, paprika, oregano, thyme, salt, and pepper. Rub the mixture onto the chicken breasts.

3. Combine the olive oil, bell peppers, red onion, zucchini, and garlic in a large mixing bowl. To coat, toss with a fork.

4. Place the chicken breasts on the grill and cook for 6 minutes. Flip the chicken and cook for an additional 6 minutes or until the chicken is cooked through.

5. Place the vegetables in a grill basket and place on the grill. Grill for 5 minutes, then flip and grill for 5 more minutes or until the vegetables are tender.

6. Drizzle the balsamic vinegar over the vegetables and stir to coat.

7. Serve the grilled chicken with the roasted vegetables on the side. Enjoy!

Snack: Apple slices with peanut butter

Ingredients:

-2 apples

-2 tablespoons of creamy peanut butter

-1 teaspoon of honey (optional)

Instructions:

1. Cut the apples into thin slices and place them on a plate.

2. Spread the peanut butter on each of the slices.

3. Drizzle the honey over the slices (optional).

4. Enjoy your apple slices with peanut butter!

CHAPTER 11

Intermittent Recipes

Breakfast

1. Oatmeal with Fruit and Nuts

Ingredients:

- 1/2 cup rolled oats

- 2/3 cup milk

- 2 tablespoons of chopped nuts (almonds, walnuts, etc.)

- 1/4 cup of mixed dried fruit (raisins, cranberries, cherries, etc.)

Instructions:

- In a medium saucepan, add oats and milk and bring to a boil over medium-high heat.

- Reduce heat to low and simmer for 4-5 minutes, stirring occasionally.

- Remove from heat and stir in the chopped nuts and dried fruit.

- Serve hot.

2. Breakfast Smoothie Bowl

Ingredients:

- 1 cup frozen berries

- 1/2 banana

- 1/2 cup plain or vanilla yogurt

- 1/2 cup almond milk

- 2 tablespoons of chia seeds

- 1 tablespoon of honey

Instructions:

- In a blender, add the frozen berries, banana, yogurt, almond milk, chia seeds, and honey.

- Blend until smooth.

- Pour into a bowl and top with your favorite toppings such as fresh fruit, nuts, or granola.

- Enjoy!

3. Egg and Cheese Sandwich

Ingredients:

- 2 slices of whole wheat bread

- 2 eggs

- 1 tablespoon of butter

- 2 slices of cheese

- Salt and pepper to taste

Instructions:

- Heat a skillet over medium heat and melt the butter.

- Crack the eggs into the skillet and cook until the whites are set.

- Place the cheese slices on top of the eggs and let them melt.

- Toast the bread in a toaster.

- Place the egg and cheese mixture on one slice of bread, top with the other slice, and season with salt and pepper.

- Enjoy!

4. Avocado Toast

Ingredients:

- 2 slices of whole wheat bread

- 1 ripe avocado

- 1 tablespoon of olive oil

- 1 teaspoon of lime juice

- 1/4 teaspoon of garlic powder

- Salt and pepper to taste

Instructions:

- Toast the bread in a toaster.

- In a medium bowl, mash the avocado and mix in the olive oil, lime juice, garlic powder, and salt and pepper.

- Spread the avocado mixture onto the toasted bread and enjoy!

5. Banana Pancakes

Ingredients:

- 1 ripe banana

- 1 egg

- 1/4 cup of almond flour

- 1/4 teaspoon of baking powder

- 1 tablespoon of almond milk

- 1/2 teaspoon of cinnamon

Instructions:

- In a medium bowl, mash the banana and mix in the egg, almond flour, baking powder, almond milk, and cinnamon.

- Heat a non-stick skillet over medium heat and spray with cooking spray.

- Pour the batter onto the skillet in circles and cook for about 2 minutes.

- Flip the pancakes and cook for another 2 minutes.

- Serve with your favorite toppings and enjoy!

6. Baked Oatmeal Cups

Ingredients:

- 2 cups of rolled oats

- 2 ripe bananas

- 1/2 cup of almond milk

- 2 tablespoons of maple syrup

- 1 teaspoon of baking powder

- 1 teaspoon of cinnamon

Instructions:

- Preheat oven to 350°F.

- In a medium bowl, mash the bananas and mix in the oats, almond milk, maple syrup, baking powder, and cinnamon.

- Grease a muffin tin with cooking spray.

- Divide the oat mixture evenly among the muffin tin wells.

- Bake for 15-20 minutes or until golden brown.

- Let cool and enjoy!

7. Yogurt Parfait

Ingredients:

- 1 cup of plain yogurt

- 1/2 cup of granola

- 1/4 cup of mixed berries

Instructions:

- In a bowl or glass, layer the yogurt, granola, and mixed berries.

- Repeat the layers until the bowl or glass is full.

- Enjoy!

8. French Toast

Ingredients:

- 2 slices of whole wheat bread

- 2 eggs

- 1/4 cup of almond milk

- 1 teaspoon of vanilla extract

- 1/2 teaspoon of cinnamon

Instructions:

- In a shallow bowl, whisk together the eggs, almond milk, vanilla extract, and cinnamon.

- Heat a skillet over medium heat and spray with cooking spray.

- Dip each slice of bread into the egg mixture, coating both sides.

- Place the dipped bread onto the skillet and cook for 2-3 minutes on each side or until golden brown.

- Serve with your favorite toppings and enjoy!

9. Breakfast Burrito

Ingredients:

- 2 eggs

- 1/4 cup of shredded cheese

- 1/4 cup of diced bell peppers

- 1/4 cup of diced onions

- 2 tablespoons of salsa

- 1 whole wheat tortilla

Instructions:

- Heat a skillet over medium heat and spray with cooking spray.

- Crack the eggs into the skillet and scramble until the whites are set.

- Add the bell peppers, onions, and salsa and cook for an additional 2-3 minutes.

- Place the egg mixture onto the tortilla and top with cheese.

- Fold the sides of the tortilla over the filling and enjoy!

10. Breakfast Burrito Bowl

Ingredients:

- 2 eggs

- 1/4 cup of cooked black beans

- 1/4 cup of cooked corn

- 1/4 cup of diced bell peppers

- 1/4 cup of diced onions

- 2 tablespoons of salsa

- 1/2 cup of cooked brown rice

Instructions:

- Heat a skillet over medium heat and spray with cooking spray.

- Crack the eggs into the skillet and scramble until the whites are set.

- Add the black beans, corn, bell peppers, onions, and salsa and cook for an additional 2-3 minutes.

- Place the egg mixture into a bowl and top with the cooked brown rice.

- Enjoy!

Lunch

1. Avocado Tuna Salad

- Prep Time: 10 minutes

Ingredients:

-1 6-ounce can of tuna, drained

-1/2 avocado, diced

-2 tablespoons of mayonnaise

-2 tablespoons of diced red onion

-1 tablespoon of lemon juice

-Salt and pepper to taste

Instructions:

-In a medium bowl, combine the tuna, avocado, mayonnaise, red onion and lemon juice.

-Mix until everything is evenly combined.

-Season with salt and pepper to taste.

-Serve over a bed of greens or in a wrap.

2. Chicken Caesar Salad Wrap

Prep Time: 10 minutes

Ingredients:

-1 cooked chicken breast, diced

-2 tablespoons of Caesar salad dressing

-2 tablespoons of diced sun-dried tomatoes

-1/4 cup of croutons

-1/4 cup of Parmesan cheese

-2 tortillas

Instructions:

-In a medium bowl, combine the chicken, Caesar dressing, sun-dried tomatoes, croutons and Parmesan cheese.

-Mix until everything is evenly combined.

-Spread the mixture evenly onto one tortilla.

-Top with the other tortilla and press down lightly.

-Cut the wrap in half and serve.

3. Egg Salad Sandwich

Prep Time: 10 minutes

Ingredients:

-2 boiled eggs, diced

-2 tablespoons of mayonnaise

-2 tablespoons of diced celery

-1 tablespoon of chopped parsley

-1 teaspoon of Dijon mustard

-Salt and pepper to taste

-2 slices of bread

Instructions:

-In a medium bowl, combine the eggs, mayonnaise, celery, parsley and Dijon mustard.

-Mix until everything is evenly combined.

-Season with salt and pepper to taste.

-Place one slice of bread with the egg salad on top.

-Top with the other slice of bread and press down lightly.

-Cut the sandwich in half and serve.

4. Quinoa Black Bean Salad

Prep Time: 10 minutes

Ingredients:

-1 cup of cooked quinoa

-1/2 cup of cooked black beans

-2 tablespoons of diced red onion

-2 tablespoons of diced bell pepper

-1 tablespoon of olive oil

-1 tablespoon of lime juice

-Salt and pepper to taste

Instructions:

-In a medium bowl, combine the quinoa, black beans, red onion, bell pepper, olive oil, and lime juice.

-Mix until everything is evenly combined.

-Season with salt and pepper to taste.

-Serve over a bed of greens or in a wrap.

5. Turkey and Hummus Wrap

Prep Time: 10 minutes

Ingredients:

-2 ounces of sliced turkey

-2 tablespoons of hummus

-2 tablespoons of diced cucumber

-2 tablespoons of diced red onion

-2 tortillas

Instructions:

-In a medium bowl, combine the turkey, hummus, cucumber and red onion.

-Mix until everything is evenly combined.

-Spread the mixture evenly onto one tortilla.

-Top with the other tortilla and press down lightly.

-Cut the wrap in half and serve.

6. Grilled Cheese Sandwich

Prep Time: 10 minutes

Ingredients:

-2 slices of bread

-2 tablespoons of butter

-2 slices of cheese

Instructions:

-Heat a skillet over medium-high heat and add the butter.

-Once the butter has melted, add the bread slices.

-Top one slice with the cheese and then place the other slice on top.

-Cook for 3-4 minutes per side, or until the cheese has melted and the bread is golden-brown.

-Cut the sandwich in half and serve.

7. Greek Yogurt Fruit Bowl

Prep Time: 10 minutes

Ingredients:

-1 cup of Greek yogurt

-1/2 cup of fresh fruit (berries, banana, etc.)

-2 tablespoons of granola

-1 tablespoon of honey (optional)

Instructions:

-In a medium bowl, add the Greek yogurt.

-Top with the fresh fruit, granola and honey (if using).

-Mix until everything is evenly combined.

-Serve immediately.

8. Egg and Avocado Toast

Prep Time: 10 minutes

Ingredients:

-2 slices of toast

-1/2 avocado, mashed

-1 boiled egg, sliced

-Salt and pepper to taste

Instructions:

-Spread the mashed avocado onto the toast slices.

-Top with the boiled egg slices.

-Season with salt and pepper to taste.

-Serve immediately.

9. Spinach and Feta Quesadilla

Prep Time: 10 minutes

Ingredients:

-2 tortillas

-1/2 cup of spinach, chopped

-2 tablespoons of feta cheese

-1 tablespoon of olive oil

Instructions:

-Heat a skillet over medium-high heat and add the olive oil.

-Once the oil is hot, add one tortilla and top with the spinach and feta cheese.

-Top with the other tortilla and press down lightly.

-Cook for 3-4 minutes per side, or until the cheese has melted and the tortilla is golden-brown.

-Cut the quesadilla in half and serve.

10. Chickpea Salad Sandwich

Prep Time: 10 minutes

Ingredients:

-1 cup of cooked chickpeas, mashed

-2 tablespoons of diced red onion

-2 tablespoons of diced celery

-2 tablespoons of mayonnaise

-2 slices of bread

Instructions:

-In a medium bowl, combine the chickpeas, red onion, celery and mayonnaise.

-Mix until everything is evenly combined.

-Spread the chickpea salad onto one slice of bread.

-Top with the other slice of bread and press down lightly.

-Cut the sandwich in half and serve.

Dinner

1. Grilled Cheese and Tomato Soup

Prep Time: 10 Minutes

Ingredients:

• 4 slices of bread

• 2 tablespoons butter

• 2 slices cheddar cheese

• 2 cups tomato soup

Instructions:

• Spread butter on one side of each slice of bread.

• Place one slice of bread butter-side-down in a hot skillet.

• Place a slice of cheese on the bread and top with the other slice of bread, butter-side-up.

• Grill each side until golden brown and the cheese is melted.

• Serve with the tomato soup.

2. Baked Salmon with Garlic Butter

Prep Time: 25 Minutes

Ingredients:

• 2 salmon fillets

• 2 tablespoons butter

• 2 cloves garlic, minced

• 2 tablespoons lemon juice

• 2 tablespoons fresh parsley, chopped

• Salt and pepper to taste

Instructions:

• Preheat oven to 375°F.

• Place salmon fillets in a greased baking dish.

• In a small saucepan, melt butter over medium heat.

• Add garlic and lemon juice and simmer for 1-2 minutes.

• Pour garlic butter over the salmon and sprinkle with parsley, salt, and pepper.

• Bake for 15 minutes or until salmon is cooked through.

3. Greek Salad

Prep Time: 15 Minutes

Ingredients:

- 2 cups romaine lettuce, chopped

- 1 cup cherry tomatoes, halved

- ½ cup feta cheese, crumbled

- ¼ cup Kalamata olives, pitted and halved

- 2 tablespoons olive oil

- 2 tablespoons red wine vinegar

- 1 teaspoon oregano

- Salt and pepper to taste

Instructions:

- In a large bowl, combine lettuce, tomatoes, feta, and olives.

- In a small bowl, whisk together olive oil, vinegar, oregano, salt, and pepper.

- Pour dressing over the salad and toss to combine.

4. Chicken Fajitas

Prep Time: 25 Minutes

Ingredients:

- 2 tablespoons olive oil

- 1 onion, sliced

- 1 bell pepper, sliced

- 1 pound boneless skinless chicken breasts, sliced

- 1 teaspoon chili powder

- 1 teaspoon cumin

- Salt and pepper to taste

- 8 flour tortillas

Instructions:

- Heat olive oil in a large skillet over medium-high heat.

- Add onion and bell pepper and cook until softened, about 5 minutes.

- Add chicken and spices and cook until chicken is cooked through, about 10 minutes.

- Serve chicken mixture in warm tortillas.

5. Macaroni and Cheese

Prep Time: 20 Minutes

Ingredients:

- 2 cups macaroni

- 2 tablespoons butter

• 2 tablespoons all-purpose flour

• 2 cups milk

• 1 teaspoon mustard powder

• 1 teaspoon garlic powder

• 1 cup cheddar cheese, shredded

• Salt and pepper to taste

Instructions:

• Cook macaroni according to package directions.

• In a large saucepan, melt butter over medium heat.

• Whisk in flour and cook for 1 minute.

• Gradually whisk in milk, mustard powder, and garlic powder.

• Simmer until sauce is thickened, about 5 minutes.

• Remove from heat and stir in cheese, salt, and pepper.

• Pour cheese sauce over cooked macaroni and stir to combine.

6. Veggie Quesadillas

Prep Time: 20 Minutes

Ingredients:

- 2 tablespoons olive oil

- 1 onion, diced

- 1 bell pepper, diced

- 2 cups mushrooms, sliced

- 4 flour tortillas

- 2 cups shredded cheese

- Salt and pepper to taste

Instructions:

- Heat olive oil in a large skillet over medium-high heat.

- Add onion, bell pepper, and mushrooms and cook until softened, about 5 minutes.

- Place a tortilla in the skillet and top with the vegetable mixture and shredded cheese.

- Top with a second tortilla and cook until cheese is melted and tortilla is golden brown, about 5 minutes.

- Cut into wedges and serve.

7. Creamy Tomato Soup

Prep Time: 15 Minutes

Ingredients:

• 2 tablespoons butter

• 1 onion, diced

• 2 cloves garlic, minced

• 2 cans diced tomatoes

• 1 cup chicken broth

• 1 cup heavy cream

• 1 teaspoon sugar

• Salt and pepper to taste

Instructions:

• Heat butter in a large pot over medium heat.

• Add onion and garlic and cook until softened, about 5 minutes.

• Add tomatoes, chicken broth, and cream and bring to a boil.

• Reduce heat and simmer for 10 minutes.

• Add sugar, salt, and pepper and stir to combine.

• Serve hot.

8. Avocado Toast

Prep Time: 10 Minutes

Ingredients:

• 2 slices of bread

• 1 avocado, mashed

• 2 tablespoons olive oil

• 1 teaspoon lemon juice

• Salt and pepper to taste

Instructions:

• Toast the bread.

• In a small bowl, mash the avocado with olive oil and lemon juice.

• Spread the mashed avocado on the toast and sprinkle with salt and pepper.

9. Spinach and Ricotta Pizza

Prep Time: 25 Minutes

Ingredients:

• 1 pizza dough

- 1 cup ricotta cheese

- 2 cups spinach, chopped

- ½ cup mozzarella cheese, shredded

- ¼ cup parmesan cheese, grated

- 2 cloves garlic, minced

- 2 tablespoons olive oil

- Salt and pepper to taste

Instructions:

- Preheat oven to 425°F.

- Roll out pizza dough and place on a baking sheet.

- In a small bowl, combine ricotta, spinach, mozzarella, parmesan, garlic, olive oil, salt, and pepper.

- Spread the cheese mixture over the pizza dough.

- Bake for 15-20 minutes or until cheese is melted and crust is golden brown.

10. Egg Salad Sandwich

Prep Time: 10 Minutes

Ingredients:

- 6 hard-boiled eggs, chopped

- ¼ cup mayonnaise

- 1 tablespoon Dijon mustard

- 1 tablespoon diced onion

- 1 teaspoon dill

- Salt and pepper to taste

- 4 slices of bread

Instructions:

- In a medium bowl, mix together eggs, mayonnaise, mustard, onion, dill, salt, and pepper.

- Spread the egg salad on the slices of bread.

- Serve.

Snacks

1. Chocolate Chip Cookie Dough Balls

Prep Time: 15 minutes

Introduction: These delicious balls of cookie dough can be enjoyed as a snack or dessert. They are made with all natural ingredients and are super quick and easy to prepare.

Ingredients:

•1 cup almond flour

•2 tablespoons coconut flour

•1/4 teaspoon fine salt

•1/4 teaspoon baking soda

•3 tablespoons coconut oil, melted

•3 tablespoons maple syrup

•1/2 teaspoon vanilla extract

•3 tablespoons chocolate chips

Preparation:

1. In a medium bowl, mix together the almond flour, coconut flour, salt and baking soda until combined.

2. Add the coconut oil, maple syrup and vanilla extract and stir until combined.

3. Fold in the chocolate chips.

4. Using your hands, form the dough into 1-inch balls and place on a parchment-lined baking sheet.

5. Place in the refrigerator for 15 minutes to firm up.

6. Enjoy!

2. Sweet Potato Fries

Prep Time: 25 minutes

Introduction: These sweet potato fries are a great snack for any time of day. They are crunchy, flavorful and packed with nutrition.

Ingredients:

•2 large sweet potatoes

•2 tablespoons olive oil

•1/2 teaspoon salt

•1/4 teaspoon black pepper

•1/4 teaspoon garlic powder

•1/4 teaspoon paprika

Preparation:

1. Preheat oven to 425 degrees F.

2. Peel and cut the sweet potatoes into 1/4-inch thick wedges.

3. Place the sweet potatoes in a large bowl and drizzle with olive oil.

4. Add the salt, black pepper, garlic powder and paprika and mix until all the potatoes are coated.

5. Place the potatoes on a baking sheet lined with parchment paper.

6. Bake for 20-25 minutes, flipping halfway through.

7. Enjoy!

3. Apple Cinnamon Muffins

Prep Time: 25 minutes

Introduction: These muffins are a delicious and healthy snack for any time of day. The combination of apples and cinnamon creates a delicious flavor.

Ingredients:

•1 cup all-purpose flour

•1 teaspoon baking powder

•1/2 teaspoon baking soda

•1/4 teaspoon salt

•1 teaspoon ground cinnamon

•1/4 cup applesauce

•1/4 cup honey

•1/4 cup melted coconut oil

•1/2 teaspoon vanilla extract

•1 large egg

•1 cup peeled, diced apples

Preparation:

1. Preheat oven to 375 degrees F.

2. In a large bowl, mix together the flour, baking powder, baking soda, salt and cinnamon.

3. In a separate bowl, mix together the applesauce, honey, coconut oil, vanilla extract and egg.

4. Add the wet ingredients to the dry ingredients and mix until just combined.

5. Fold in the diced apples.

6. Spoon the batter into a greased muffin tin, filling each cup about 3/4 of the way full.

7. Bake for 20-25 minutes or until a toothpick inserted in the center comes out clean.

8. Enjoy!

4. Cucumber Avocado Toast

Prep Time: 15 minutes

Introduction: This toast is a delicious and healthy snack. It is packed with protein, fiber and healthy fats from the avocado.

Ingredients:

•2 slices whole wheat bread

•1/2 avocado

•1/2 cucumber, thinly sliced

•1/4 teaspoon salt

•1/4 teaspoon black pepper

•1/4 teaspoon garlic powder

•1/4 teaspoon paprika

•1 tablespoon olive oil

Preparation:

1. Toast the bread until golden brown.

2. Mash the avocado with a fork and spread on the toast.

3. Top with the thinly sliced cucumber.

4. Sprinkle with the salt, black pepper, garlic powder and paprika.

5. Drizzle with the olive oil.

6. Enjoy!

5. Peanut Butter Banana Bites

Prep Time: 5 minutes

Introduction: These bites are a delicious and healthy snack. They are packed with protein and fiber and can be enjoyed on the go.

Ingredients:

•2 bananas

•1/4 cup peanut butter

•2 tablespoons honey

•1/4 cup chopped peanuts

Preparation:

1. Slice the bananas into 1/2-inch thick slices.

2. Spread the peanut butter and honey on the slices.

3. Sprinkle with the chopped peanuts.

4. Serve or store in an airtight container.

5. Enjoy!

6. Kale Chips

Prep Time: 20 minutes

Introduction: These crunchy kale chips are a great snack for any time of day. They are packed with vitamins and minerals and are super easy to prepare.

Ingredients:

•1 bunch kale

•2 tablespoons olive oil

•1/2 teaspoon salt

•1/4 teaspoon black pepper

•1/4 teaspoon garlic powder

•1/4 teaspoon paprika

Preparation:

1. Preheat oven to 350 degrees F.

2. Wash and dry the kale leaves and remove the stems.

3. Cut the leaves into 1-inch pieces.

4. Place the kale pieces in a large bowl and drizzle with olive oil.

5. Sprinkle with the salt, black pepper, garlic powder and paprika and mix until all the kale is coated.

6. Spread the kale on a baking sheet lined with parchment paper.

7. Bake for 15-20 minutes or until the chips are crispy.

8. Enjoy!

7. Carrot Hummus

Prep Time: 10 minutes

Introduction: This carrot hummus is a delicious and nutritious snack. It is packed with fiber and plant-based protein and is super quick and easy to prepare.

Ingredients:

•1 can chickpeas, drained and rinsed

•2 carrots, chopped

•2 cloves garlic, minced

•1/4 cup tahini

•3 tablespoons olive oil

•1 tablespoon lemon juice

•1/2 teaspoon ground cumin

•1/4 teaspoon salt

Preparation:

1. In a food processor, combine the chickpeas, carrots, garlic, tahini, olive oil, lemon juice, cumin, and salt.

2. Process until smooth and creamy.

3. Serve with vegetables or crackers.

4. Enjoy!

8. Popcorn Trail Mix

Prep Time: 5 minutes

Introduction: This trail mix is a great snack to have on hand for when you're on the go. It's packed with nutrition and is super easy to make.

Ingredients:

•2 cups air-popped popcorn

•1/2 cup dried cranberries

•1/2 cup chopped almonds

•1/4 cup sunflower seeds

•1/4 cup pumpkin seeds

•1/4 cup dark chocolate chips

Preparation:

1. Place the popcorn, cranberries, almonds, sunflower seeds, pumpkin seeds and dark chocolate chips in a bowl.

2. Mix until combined.

3. Serve or store in an airtight container.

4. Enjoy!

9. Baked Apple Chips

Prep Time: 25 minutes

Introduction: These delicious apple chips are a great way to satisfy your sweet tooth. They are crunchy and healthy and are super easy to make.

Ingredients:

•2 apples, cored and thinly sliced

•1 teaspoon ground cinnamon

•1/4 teaspoon ground nutmeg

•1/4 teaspoon ground ginger

•1/4 teaspoon ground allspice

•1/4 teaspoon salt

•1 tablespoon maple syrup

Preparation:

1. Preheat oven to 250 degrees F.

2. Line a baking sheet with parchment paper and place the apple slices on it.

3. Sprinkle with the cinnamon, nutmeg, ginger, allspice and salt.

4. Drizzle with the maple syrup.

5. Bake for 20-25 minutes or until the chips are crispy.

6. Enjoy!

10. Zucchini Fritters

Prep Time: 25 minutes

Introduction: These tasty fritters are a great snack for any time of day. They are packed with nutrition and are super easy to make.

Ingredients:

•2 large zucchinis, grated

•1/2 cup all-purpose flour

•1 teaspoon baking powder

•1/2 teaspoon salt

•1/4 teaspoon black pepper

•1/4 teaspoon garlic powder

•1/4 teaspoon paprika

•1 egg, beaten

•1/4 cup olive oil

Preparation:

1. In a large bowl, mix together the grated zucchini, flour, baking powder, salt, black pepper, garlic powder and paprika.

2. Add the beaten egg and mix until combined.

3. Heat the olive oil in a large skillet over medium heat.

4. Drop the zucchini mixture by the tablespoonful into the hot oil and flatten slightly.

5. Cook for 2-3 minutes per side or until golden brown.

6. Transfer to a paper towel-lined plate to absorb excess oil.

7. Enjoy!

Desserts

1. Coconut Date Bars:

Introduction: These Coconut Date Bars are made with almond flour, dates, and coconut flakes for a delicious snack that is loaded with healthy fats and natural sweetness.

Ingredients:

- 2 cups almond flour

- 1 tsp baking powder

- 1/2 tsp salt

- 1/2 cup coconut oil, melted

- 1/2 cup honey

- 1 cup pitted dates, chopped

- 1/2 cup unsweetened shredded coconut

Preparation:

1. Preheat oven to 350°F.

2. In a medium bowl, mix together the almond flour, baking powder, and salt.

3. In a separate bowl, mix together the melted coconut oil, honey, and chopped dates.

4. Slowly add the wet ingredients to the dry ingredients and mix until combined.

5. Transfer the dough to a greased 9x13 inch baking pan and press down evenly.

6. Sprinkle the shredded coconut over the top of the dough and lightly press down.

7. Bake for 20 minutes or until golden brown.

8. Allow to cool before cutting into bars.

Prep Time: 10 minutes

2. Chocolate Coconut Bites:

Introduction: These Chocolate Coconut Bites are a delicious and easy to make treat that is perfect for any occasion.

Ingredients:

- 1/2 cup dark chocolate chips

- 1/2 cup shredded coconut

- 1/4 cup honey

- 2 tbsp coconut oil

- 1/4 tsp sea salt

Preparation:

1. In a small saucepan, melt the dark chocolate chips over low heat.

2. Once the chocolate is melted, add the shredded coconut, honey, coconut oil, and sea salt. Mix until combined.

3. Line a baking sheet with parchment paper.

4. Drop spoonfuls of the mixture onto the parchment paper and spread out into small circles.

5. Place in the refrigerator for 30 minutes or until hardened.

6. Serve chilled or at room temperature.

Prep Time: 10 minutes

3. Almond Butter Fudge:

Introduction: This Almond Butter Fudge is made with almond butter, honey, and dark chocolate for a delicious and easy to make treat.

Ingredients:

- 1 cup almond butter

- 1/4 cup honey

- 1/4 cup dark chocolate chips

- 1/4 tsp sea salt

Preparation:

1. In a small saucepan, melt the dark chocolate chips over low heat.

2. Once the chocolate is melted, add the almond butter, honey, and sea salt. Mix until combined.

3. Line a baking sheet with parchment paper.

4. Spread the mixture onto the parchment paper and spread out into a thin layer.

5. Place in the refrigerator for 30 minutes or until hardened.

6. Cut into small cubes and serve chilled or at room temperature.

Prep Time: 10 minutes

4. Date Cashew Balls:

Introduction: These Date Cashew Balls are made with dates, cashews, and coconut for a delicious and nutrient-packed snack.

Ingredients:

- 2 cups pitted dates

- 1 cup unsalted cashews

- 1/4 cup shredded coconut

- 1/4 tsp sea salt

Preparation:

1. In a food processor, combine the dates, cashews, shredded coconut, and sea salt. Blend until the mixture is combined and forms a sticky dough.

2. Using a spoon or your hands, form the mixture into small balls and transfer to a parchment paper-lined baking sheet.

3. Place the balls in the refrigerator for 30 minutes or until hardened.

4. Serve chilled or at room temperature.

Prep Time: 10 minutes

5. No Bake Chocolate Peanut Butter Oat Bars:

Introduction: These No Bake Chocolate Peanut Butter Oat Bars are made with oats, peanut butter, and dark chocolate for a delicious and easy to make snack.

Ingredients:

- 2 cups rolled oats

- 1/2 cup peanut butter

- 1/2 cup honey

- 1/2 cup dark chocolate chips

- 1/4 tsp sea salt

Preparation:

1. In a medium bowl, mix together the rolled oats, peanut butter, honey, and sea salt.

2. Line a 9x13 inch baking pan with parchment paper.

3. Spread the mixture evenly into the pan and press down using a spoon.

4. Melt the dark chocolate chips in a small saucepan over low heat.

5. Once the chocolate is melted, spread it evenly over the top of the oat mixture.

6. Place in the refrigerator for 30 minutes or until hardened.

7. Cut into bars and serve chilled or at room temperature.

Prep Time: 10 minutes

6. Apple Pie Bites:

Introduction: These Apple Pie Bites are made with apples, cinnamon, and almond flour for a delicious and healthy snack.

Ingredients:

- 2 apples, peeled and diced

- 2 tbsp almond flour

- 2 tsp cinnamon

- 1/4 cup honey

Preparation:

1. Preheat oven to 350°F.

2. In a medium bowl, mix together the diced apples, almond flour, cinnamon, and honey.

3. Line a baking sheet with parchment paper.

4. Scoop spoonfuls of the mixture onto the parchment paper and lightly press down.

5. Bake for 15 minutes or until golden brown.

6. Allow to cool before serving.

Prep Time: 10 minutes

7. No Bake Almond Coconut Bars:

Introduction: These No Bake Almond Coconut Bars are made with almond butter, coconut flakes, and dark chocolate for an easy and delicious treat.

Ingredients:

- 1 cup almond butter

- 1/2 cup shredded coconut

- 1/2 cup honey

- 1/2 cup dark chocolate chips

- 1/4 tsp sea salt

Preparation:

1. Line a 9x13 inch baking pan with parchment paper.

2. In a medium bowl, mix together the almond butter, shredded coconut, honey, and sea salt.

3. Spread the mixture evenly into the pan and press down using a spoon.

4. Melt the dark chocolate chips in a small saucepan over low heat.

5. Once the chocolate is melted, spread it evenly over the top of the almond mixture.

6. Place in the refrigerator for 30 minutes or until hardened.

7. Cut into bars and serve chilled or at room temperature.

Prep Time: 10 minutes

8. No Bake Chocolate Coconut Cookies:

Introduction: These No Bake Chocolate Coconut Cookies are made with coconut flakes, almond butter, and dark chocolate for a delicious and easy to make snack.

Ingredients:

- 1 cup shredded coconut

- 1/2 cup almond butter

- 1/2 cup honey

- 1/2 cup dark chocolate chips

- 1/4 tsp sea salt

Preparation:

1. Line a baking sheet with parchment paper.

2. In a medium bowl, mix together the shredded coconut, almond butter, honey, and sea salt.

3. Drop spoonfuls of the mixture onto the parchment paper and spread out into small circles.

4. Melt the dark chocolate chips in a small saucepan over low heat.

5. Once the chocolate is melted, spread it evenly over the top of the coconut mixture.

6. Place in the refrigerator for 30 minutes or until hardened.

7. Serve chilled or at room temperature.

Prep Time: 10 minutes

9. No Bake Peanut Butter Chia Bars:

Introduction: These No Bake Peanut Butter Chia Bars are made with peanut butter, chia seeds, and coconut for a delicious and nutrient-packed snack.

Ingredients:

- 1 cup peanut butter

- 1/2 cup chia seeds

- 1/2 cup shredded coconut

- 1/4 cup honey

- 1/4 tsp sea salt

Preparation:

1. Line a 9x13 inch baking pan with parchment paper.

2. In a medium bowl, mix together the peanut butter, chia seeds, shredded coconut, honey, and sea salt.

3. Spread the mixture evenly into the pan and press down using a spoon.

4. Place in the refrigerator for 30 minutes or until hardened.

5. Cut into bars and serve chilled or at room temperature.

Prep Time: 10 minutes

10. No Bake Trail Mix Bars:

Introduction: These No Bake Trail Mix Bars are made with oats, dried fruit, and nuts for a delicious and portable snack.

Ingredients:

- 2 cups old-fashioned rolled oats

- 1/2 cup dried fruit of your choice (raisins, cranberries, etc.)

- 1/2 cup nuts of your choice (almonds, walnuts, etc.)

- 1/4 cup honey

- 1/4 tsp sea salt

Preparation:

1. Line a 9x13 inch baking pan with parchment paper.

2. In a medium bowl, mix together the rolled oats, dried fruit, nuts, honey, and sea salt.

3. Spread the mixture evenly into the pan and press down using a spoon.

4. Place in the refrigerator for 30 minutes or until hardened.

5. Cut into bars and serve chilled or at room temperature.

Prep Time: 10 minutes

Smoothies

1) Peach-Banana Smoothie:

This refreshing smoothie is a blend of sweet peaches and bananas with a hint of tartness from the lemon juice. It's a great way to kickstart your morning or cool off after a hot day. Prep time: 5 minutes.

Ingredients:

• 2 ripe bananas, peeled and sliced

• 1 cup frozen peach slices

- ½ cup plain Greek yogurt

- 1 tablespoon honey

- ¼ cup orange juice

- 1 tablespoon freshly squeezed lemon juice

Preparation:

1. Place all ingredients in a blender and blend until smooth.

2. Pour into two glasses and enjoy.

2) Tropical Green Smoothie:

A tropical green smoothie with a blend of pineapple, mango, and banana with a hint of lime to give it an extra zing. Prep time: 5 minutes.

Ingredients:

- ½ cup fresh pineapple

- ½ cup mango

- 1 banana

- 2 cups spinach

- 1 tablespoon lime juice

- ½ cup almond milk

Preparation:

1. Place all ingredients in a blender and blend until smooth.

2. Pour into two glasses and enjoy.

3) Chocolate Peanut Butter Smoothie:

A creamy smoothie that is packed with protein and chocolatey goodness. Prep time: 5 minutes.

Ingredients:

• 1 banana

• ½ cup plain Greek yogurt

• 2 tablespoons peanut butter

• 1 tablespoon cocoa powder

• ½ cup almond milk

Preparation:

1. Place all ingredients in a blender and blend until smooth.

2. Pour into two glasses and enjoy.

4) Blueberry Banana Smoothie:

A creamy smoothie with a hint of tartness from the blueberries and sweetness from the banana. Prep time: 5 minutes.

Ingredients:

• 1 banana

• ½ cup fresh or frozen blueberries

• ½ cup plain Greek yogurt

• 1 tablespoon honey

• ½ cup almond milk

Preparation:

1. Place all ingredients in a blender and blend until smooth.

2. Pour into two glasses and enjoy.

5) Strawberry-Kiwi Smoothie:

A sweet and tangy smoothie with a blend of strawberries and kiwis. Prep time: 5 minutes.

Ingredients:

• 1 banana

• ½ cup fresh or frozen strawberries

- ½ cup fresh or frozen kiwi

- ½ cup plain Greek yogurt

- ½ cup almond milk

Preparation:

1. Place all ingredients in a blender and blend until smooth.

2. Pour into two glasses and enjoy.

6) Mango-Avocado Smoothie:

A creamy and refreshing smoothie with a tropical twist. Prep time: 5 minutes.

Ingredients:

- 1 banana

- ½ cup fresh or frozen mango

- ½ avocado

- ½ cup plain Greek yogurt

- ½ cup almond milk

Preparation:

1. Place all ingredients in a blender and blend until smooth.

2. Pour into two glasses and enjoy.

7) Pineapple-Coconut Smoothie:

A refreshing and tropical smoothie with sweet pineapple and creamy coconut. Prep time: 5 minutes.

Ingredients:

• 1 banana

• ½ cup fresh or frozen pineapple

• ½ cup coconut milk

• 1 tablespoon honey

• ½ cup almond milk

Preparation:

1. Place all ingredients in a blender and blend until smooth.

2. Pour into two glasses and enjoy.

8) Acai Berry Smoothie:

A superfood smoothie with the antioxidant-packed acai berry. Prep time: 5 minutes.

Ingredients:

• 1 banana

• 1 cup frozen acai berry

- ½ cup plain Greek yogurt

- 1 tablespoon honey

- ½ cup almond milk

Preparation:

1. Place all ingredients in a blender and blend until smooth.

2. Pour into two glasses and enjoy.

9) Mixed Berry Smoothie: A refreshing smoothie with a blend of raspberries, blueberries, and strawberries. Prep time: 5 minutes.

Ingredients:

- 1 banana

- ½ cup fresh or frozen raspberries

- ½ cup fresh or frozen blueberries

- ½ cup fresh or frozen strawberries

- ½ cup plain Greek yogurt

- ½ cup almond milk

Preparation:

1. Place all ingredients in a blender and blend until smooth.

2. Pour into two glasses and enjoy.

10) Apple-Cinnamon Smoothie:

An autumn-inspired smoothie with the flavors of apples and cinnamon. Prep time: 5 minutes.

Ingredients:

• 1 banana

• 1 cup diced apples

• ½ teaspoon ground cinnamon

• ½ cup plain Greek yogurt

• ½ cup almond milk

Preparation:

1. Place all ingredients in a blender and blend until smooth.

2. Pour into two glasses and enjoy.